Getting that fit and sexy Body

MATTHEW BAMIGBOSE

ISBN:9798360061854

DEDICATION

This book is dedicated to the beautiful females who need that extra confidence tips and guide to equally getting a beautiful and sexy body.

CONTENTS

ACKNOWLEDGMENTS

I want to specially thank the people who made this book a possibility to publish. Not forgetting my family for creating that atmosphere to write successfully.

EXERCISE BASICS

Physical activity is defined as any movement that requires you to contract your muscles. Housekeeping, gardening, walking, and climbing the stairs are all examples of physical activity.

The Basics

Exercise is a type of physical activity that is planned and performed with the goal of improving fitness or other health benefits. Exercising at a health club, swimming, cycling, running, and sports such as golf and tennis are all examples of physical activity.

How can you tell whether an action is moderate or vigorous in intensity? It's moderate if you can talk while performing it. It's vigorous if you have to stop to catch your breath after only a few words.

A game of doubles tennis would likely be moderate in intensity, depending on your fitness level, whereas a singles game could be more vigorous. Furthermore, ballroom dancing is considered moderate, whereas aerobic dancing is considered vigorous. Once again, it's not just your choice of activity, but also how much effort it requires.

An ideal exercise regimen would include elements that improve each of these components:

Cardiovascular endurance. Improve your respiratory endurance (your ability to perform aerobics) by brisk walking, jogging, running, cycling, swimming, jumping rope, rowing, or cross-country skiing. As you reach your distance or intensity level goals, raise them or switch to a different action to keep yourself challenged.

Muscular power. Lifting weights, either free weights like barbells and dumbbells or lifting machines, is the most efficient way to improve muscular strength.

Muscular endurance. Better your endurance with calisthenics (conditioning exercises), weight training, and actions like running or swimming.

Flexibleness. Improve your flexibility by performing stretching exercises as part of your exercise routine or by participating in a stretching-focused discipline such as yoga or pilates.

Although a physically active lifestyle can handle all of these fitness factors, an exercise program can help you achieve even greater benefits.

Increasing the total amount of physical activity in your daily life is a great place to start, such as parking a couple of blocks away from your destination to get in some walking. To truly achieve fitness goals, however, you'll need to incorporate structured, vigorous actions into your schedule to help you achieve even more fitness and health goals.

SET YOUR GOAL AND STICK TO IT

Starting or returning to a workout routine entails more than just planning your exercises and joining a gym. In fact, it is entirely possible to join a gym and never go, even if the monthly payments appear on your bank statement. I understand because I've done it a few times in my life. Sticking to your goals necessitates a few mental tricks to keep you going, centered, and motivated.

Keep Going

Momentum is an essential component of uniform exercise. It's normal to have weeks when everything goes perfectly: you do all your exercises, eat like a health nut, and start thinking, 'I might be able to finish this!'

Then 'it' manifests itself.

It could be a vacation, an illness, or something else that throws you off guard. Returning is always difficult, partly because you've lost your momentum. We know that an object at rest tends to stay at rest, so getting moving again is the only way to get your momentum moving.

Instead of focusing on making up for lost time with intense exercises, focus on simply getting some exercise in. Plan your workouts for the week and consider yourself successful just for showing up.

Purchase something small for yourself, such as a new pair of running shoes or an exceptional pair of gym shorts. If you're having trouble getting back into it, buy a new outfit or add a few new songs to your MP3 player to give yourself something to look forward to.

Make an appointment to exercise with a friend or contact your gym to schedule a free consultation with a personal trainer. Even if you do not sign up, getting back into an exercise routine may be exactly what you need.

Do something completely different if the thought of returning to boring gym exercises makes you want to die. Register for a local belly dance class or visit that new yoga studio. A change of scenery and a new activity may refresh and revitalize you.

Consider this: you're at a party and have promised yourself that you won't gorge yourself on the buffet. Then you notice a massive platter of the most beautiful cheese you've ever seen. Many hours later, as your cheese hangover begins, you resolve to make amends with a long workout the next day.

There are some drawbacks to this approach: first, you can't undo what you ate the night before; second, killing yourself with exercise isn't a good solution because it makes you hate exercise even more.

If you're focused on yesterday's mistakes, many of your decisions will be based on guilt and shame rather than what you really want (and need) to do to achieve your goals. True change comes from daily choices, and becoming mindful and basing your choices on what you need now (rather than what you did or did not do yesterday) will make your exercise life much more bearable.

GET YOUR EXERCISE PLAN TOGETHER

Taking the time to sit down and create a concrete schedule is the critical first step toward achieving the body you desire. Following that comes the difficult task of sticking to it each week, but that's a different topic for another day; for now, let's just focus on creating a workout schedule.

Putting A Plan Together

Sit down with a weekly calendar and decide how many days of the week you're willing to exercise.
Decide on the type of workout that you want to do. Cardiovascular exercise, for example, will help you lose fat while lifting weights will help you build muscle.
Commit to exercising according to your plan. This is the most important step.

Stick to your schedule for at least one month. The progress you'll see after four weeks should be sufficient to keep you motivated.

Cardiovascular workout

• Make time in your schedule for 30-minute workouts. Most people can get by with 30 minutes of exercise per day.
• Select a type of cardiovascular workout for a specific day of the week.

Jogging, bicycling, and swimming are all effective forms of cardiovascular exercise that can be done on a treadmill or stair-climbing machine.

- Warm up and actively stretch for five minutes before beginning any activity.

- Perform a 20-minute moderate-intensity workout.

- Finish with a five-minute cool down.

- Adjust your schedule to accommodate longer workout periods if possible.

Stick to your plans.

Weights

- Allow thirty to sixty minutes for weight training sessions. If you don't spend too much time socializing or resting during your workout, you can get a great session of lifting in. Rest no longer than sixty seconds between sets.
- Begin with total-body workouts that

target each major muscle group (upper body, lower body and back). The importance of balanced development cannot be overstated.

• As you gain experience as a lifter, divide your workouts. This will allow you to better focus on specific muscle groups and areas. Chest and triceps, back and biceps, shoulder and legs are the basic splits that target each major muscle group.

• Allow your muscles to recover between sessions. Allow at least one day between sessions for each muscle group. Muscles cannot grow unless they are given time to rest and heal.

• Tailor your agenda to best meet your objectives.

• Stick to your workout routine.

MAKE SURE TO WARM UP

During training and racing, many athletes warm up and cool down on a regular basis. A proper warm-up may increase blood flow to the working muscle, resulting in less muscle stiffness, a lower risk of injury, and improved performance. Warming up also helps with physiologic and psychological preparation.

Warm Up

Advantages of a Suitable Warm Up:
Modified Muscle Temperature - Temperature increases within muscles

used during a warm-up routine. A warmed-up muscle contracts more forcefully and relaxes more quickly. Speed and strength can both be increased in this manner. Similarly, the likelihood of pulling a muscle and causing trauma is much lower.

Modified Body Temperature - This improves muscle elasticity while also lowering the risk of strains and pulls.

Blood vessels enlarge, lowering resistance to blood flow and putting less strain on the heart.

Better Efficient Cooling - By activating the body's heat-dissipation mechanisms (effective sweating), an athlete can cool quickly and avoid overheating early in the event or race.

Modified Blood Temperature - As blood flows through the muscles, its temperature rises. As blood temperature rises, the binding of oxygen to hemoglobin decreases, making oxygen more readily available to working muscles, potentially improving

endurance.
Improved Range of Motion - A joint's range of motion is altered.

Hormonal Changes - Your body increases the production of various hormones that regulate energy production. During warm-up, this hormonal balance makes more carbs and fatty acids available for energy production.

Mental Preparation - The warm-up is also an excellent time to mentally prepare for an event by clearing the mind, improving centering, critiquing skills, and technique. Favorable imagery can also help the athlete relax and concentrate.

Typical Warm up exercises include:
Gradually increase the intensity of your chosen sport. This makes use of a sport's specific skills and is also known

as a related warm-up. For runners, the idea is to jog for a while, then add a few sprints to the routine to engage all muscle fibers.

Incorporate motions unrelated to your sport, such as calisthenics or flexibility exercises, gradually and steadily. Ball players frequently warm up with exercises that are unrelated to their sport.

Which should I go with? To avoid injury, stretch a muscle after it has experienced a change in blood flow and temperature. Stretching a cold muscle may increase the risk of strains and tears.

So, before stretching, do a gentle aerobic workout. Stretching is best done after a workout when your muscles are warm and pliable due to increased blood flow. Make sure that your warm-up is gradual and that it targets the muscles that will be strained during the workout.

Remember that the perfect warm-up

is a highly personal process that can only be attained through practice, experimentation, and experience. Warm up in various ways and intensities until you find what works best for you.

INCORPORATE CARDIO TRAINING

With a large proportion of Americans being overweight, it's clear that many of us are not following the most recent exercise guidelines, which recommend up to an hour of exercise per day. There was no doubt a collective groan when people realized they'd have to find an hour every day to do something they couldn't seem to find five minutes for. How important are these guidelines, and what can you do to incorporate them into your life?

Cardio Basics

Before we begin, you should understand why it is so important. Cardiovascular exercise simply means engaging in an activity that raises your heart rate to the point where you're working but can still talk (also known as, in your Target Heart Rate). Here's why cardio is so important:

It's one way to burn off calories and help you slim down

It makes your heart strong so that it doesn't have to work as grueling to pump blood

It step-ups your lung capacity

It helps bring down risk of heart attack, elevated cholesterol, hypertension and diabetes

It makes you feel great

It aids you in sleeping better

It helps bring down tension

I could go on all day, however you get

the point

Bottom line: if you want to lose weight and reduce stress, you must engage in cardio exercise.

The first move is to think about what kinds of activities you'd like to do. The trick is to think about what's available to you, what fits your personality, and what you'd feel comfortable incorporating into your life.

Running, bicycling, hiking, and walking are all excellent outdoor activities. If you enjoy working out in the gym, you'll have access to stationary bicycles, elliptical trainers, treadmills, row machines, stair masters, and other equipment.

There are numerous first-rate workout videos to try for the home exerciser, and you don't need much equipment to get an excellent home cardio workout.

Keep in mind that you may not yet know what type of activity you enjoy. That's all part of the learning process, so don't be afraid to try something and, if it doesn't work, try something else.

Almost any activity will work as long as it requires a motion that gets your heart rate into your Target Zone. Remember: There is no such thing as the "most proficient" cardio exercise. Anything that you enjoy and gets your heart rate up will suffice.

It's not so much what you do as it is how hard you work. Any exercise can be difficult if you make it so.

Do something you enjoy. If you despise gym workouts, avoid using a treadmill. If you enjoy socializing, consider sports, group fitness, exercising with a friend, or joining a walking club.

Choose something that you can see yourself doing at least three times per week.

Be adaptable and don't be afraid to branch out once you've gotten into a routine with exercise.

USE WEIGHTS

Lifting weights is one of the most important things you can do if you want to lose fat or change your body. Diet and cardio are equally important, but when it comes to changing the way your body looks, weight training comes out on top.

Lifting Basics

If you've been putting off starting a strength training program, knowing that lifting weights can:

Assist in increasing your metabolism. Muscle burns a lot of calories, so the more muscle you have, the more calories you'll burn off throughout the day.
Fortify bones, particularly crucial for women
Make you stronger and better muscular endurance
Help you prevent injuries
Better your confidence and self-pride
Better coordination and balance

Getting started with strength training can be difficult—what exercises can you do? How many sets and reps are there? How much lifting is involved? The routine you choose will be determined by your fitness goals, as well as the tools you have available and the amount of time you have available for exercise.

If you're starting your own program, you'll need to understand some fundamental strength training principles. These guidelines will teach you how to use appropriate weight, determine your sets and reps, and ensure you're always progressing in your workouts.

To build muscle, you must use more resistance than your muscles are accustomed to. This is critical because the more you do, the more your body can do, so you should increase your workload to avoid plateaus. In layman's terms, this means you should be lifting enough weight to complete the desired number of reps. You should be able to complete your final rep with difficulty but also with good form.

To avoid plateaus (or adaptation), you must increase your intensity on a regular basis. You can accomplish this by increasing the amount of weight lifted, changing your sets/reps, changing the exercises, and changing the type of resistance. You are able to make these alterations on a weekly or monthly basis.

Specificity. This principle implies that you should train for your goal. That is, if you want to increase your strength, your workout should be tailored to that goal (for example, train with heavier weights closer to your 1 RM (1 rep max)). To lose weight, try a variety of rep ranges that target different muscle fibers.

Rest days are just as important as workout days. Your muscles grow and change during these rest periods, so avoid working the same muscle groups two days in a row.

Before you begin creating your routine, keep the following points in mind:

Always warm up before beginning to lift weights. This helps to warm up your muscles and prevents injury. Warm up with light cardio or a light set of each exercise before progressing to heavier weights.

Slowly raise and lower your weights. Lift the weight without using momentum. If you have to swing to get the weight up, you're probably using too much weight.

Don't hold your breath, and make sure you're using your entire range of motion throughout the motion.

Straighten your back. Maintain your balance and protect your spine by paying attention to your posture and using your abs in every motion.

EAT HEALTHY

Healthy eating isn't about following strict nutrition guidelines, remaining unrealistically thin, or depriving yourself of foods you enjoy. Instead, it's about feeling good, having more energy, keeping your mood stable, and staying as healthy as possible—all of which can be achieved by learning a few nutrition basics and implementing them in a way that works for you. You can broaden your healthy food options and learn how to plan ahead of time to produce and maintain a tasty, healthy diet.

Good Habits

Consider planning a healthy diet as a series of small, manageable steps rather than one large, drastic change to increase your chances of success. You'll have a healthy diet sooner than you think if you approach the changes gradually and with dedication.

Rather than obsessing over calorie counts or portion sizes, think about your diet in terms of color, variety, and freshness.

It should be easier to make healthy choices this way. Concentrate on finding foods you enjoy and simple recipes that use a few fresh ingredients. Your diet will gradually become healthier and more delicious.

Begin slowly and gradually change your eating habits. Trying to change your diet overnight is neither realistic nor wise. Changing everything at once frequently leads to cheating or quitting your new eating plan.

Make small changes, such as adding a salad (full of different colored vegetables) to your diet once a day or switching from butter to olive oil when cooking. You can continue to add healthier options to your diet as your small changes become habit.

Every change you make to improve your diet is significant. To have a healthy diet, you don't have to be perfect or give up all of your favorite foods.

Long-term goals include feeling better, having more energy, and lowering the risk of cancer and disease. Don't let your missteps derail you—every healthy food choice you make counts.

THE BENEFITS TO A HEALTHY LIFESTYLE OTHER THAN LOOKING GREAT

The first benefit of leading a healthy lifestyle is that you will most likely live a longer and healthier life. If you have a family to support, this is critical because you will be there for them both financially and emotionally.

If you have a child, I'm sure they'll want their parents to be there for them.

Parents have the pleasure of raising their children and witnessing their development from tot to early childhood years and all the way to maturity.

As a parent, you'll get to spend time with your grandchildren and even watch them grow.

Advantages

Another advantage of leading a healthy lifestyle is that you will be more vibrant and energetic. You'll have more pep in your step. This will allow you to be more active and accomplish more. This will allow you to have a more positive attitude in life and will benefit your physical, emotional, and mental health.

It will allow you to be more productive at both home and work. You will have fewer sick days at work, making you a more productive employee. If you own a business, increased productivity may make it more profitable. Overall, increased productivity could result in significant financial dividends for you in the future.

You'll look and feel better overall. You'll have a much better outlook on life. It will pay off handsomely in terms of your physical, emotional, and mental health in the long run. It will relieve tension and stress. It will also ease and reduce your chances of developing a depressive disorder or becoming depressed all the time because you will feel better about yourself and have a more positive frame of mind.

It is a type of preventive health care and medicine. It will aid in the prevention of heart disease, cancer, and a variety of other debilitating diseases.

The best is saved for last. One of the most significant advantages of leading a healthy lifestyle is the amount of money you will save. When you're in good health, you'll;

• Spend less time and money on doctor visits.

• Save money on prescriptions.

• Fewer, if any, hospital visits

• Reduce the risk of out-of-control medical expenses, which are one of the leading causes of bankruptcy and financial ruin.

Regrettably, very few people recognize and comprehend the financial benefits of leading a healthy lifestyle.

So these are the benefits of a healthy lifestyle and how to live a healthy lifestyle in general.

WRAPPING UP

Remember that there's more to having a beautiful body than just using effective wellness products. You must be on a total preventative healthcare and wellness program that includes diet, nutrition (ensuring that your body receives the necessary nutrients), and exercise.

ABOUT THE AUTHOR

Matthew Ademola Bamigbose, who comes from a family of six. He hails and lives Lagos, Nigeria.
Matthew is a reserved person to those who don't know him and a menace to the ones that actually know him.
His main hobbies are reading and watching movies mostly k-drama contents, I know right!
He has a degree in psychology and political science

www.ingramcontent.com/pod-product-compliance
Lightning Source LLC
LaVergne TN
LVHW020526160826
845677LV00015B/3928

* 9 7 9 8 3 6 0 0 6 1 8 5 4 *